CONTENTS

INTRODUCTION
CHAPTER 1. WHAT IS THE WHOLE 30 DIET?

The Whole 30 diet is a relatively new monthly cleansing program. It is assumed that following this diet can provide a "reset" of metabolism and change the person's attitude toward food.

The program was developed based on the assumption that some product groups have a very negative impact on the health and physical endurance of a person. And therefore, if you exclude these foods from the diet, you can significantly improve your health. Both physical and mental.

The main goal of many people following the Whole 30 diet is losing weight. However, the program offers more than the usual weight loss. With its help, you can understand what products are specifically harmful to you.

For different people, the list of intolerable foods may be somewhat different. To me, the appeal of Whole 30 is that this experiment does not go beyond common sense if to compare with the other diets. I mean, of course, your skin does get better, and you generally feel and look much healthier after you quit sugar for a month. Of course, you feel full of energy after you don't smoke or drink alcohol. And of course, you experience significant health improvement after you stop consuming gluten. After all, it is not magic but pure logic.

The first step to following a whole foods diet is understanding what it means. To put it plain and straightforward, it involves filling a majority of your diet with foods that are not processed or refined and come directly from plants. They are foods that are as close as possible to their sources and are completely unmodified. **Whole 30 is pretty much a hardcore version of the Paleo diet.**

How the diet works

The idea behind the whole foods diet system is simple. The purpose is to research how the food you eat affects your body and its reactions. First, you eliminate certain foods and then reinstate them slowly after the 30-day diet is up.

Try and watch the reaction of your body. In this way, you can clearly identify which products are not useful for you. Honey may be the culprit when it comes to your runny nose; milk may be behind your stomach trouble.

The details can seem confusing — for example, from all legumes, you can eat just green beans. Also, you can eat almonds, but peanuts are out of the Whole 30 food list. Take it easy; it's not as complicated as it seems. By the way, you do not have to eat a 100% organic diet to follow the program; that is an entirely different topic. This is not to say that your entire foods cannot be organic; it is just not a prerequisite to qualify as full or natural.

Apparently, organic or locally grown food could provide you with the added benefit of eliminating harmful toxins and chemicals, which can further the health benefit of eating whole foods. So, be careful and read products labels.

To help you with your Whole 30 Vegetarian challenge, here's a step-by-step guide to all the foods you can and can't eat during the 30 days.

Whole : Vegetarian Approach

For those who follow the vegetarian lifestyle, Whole 30 is particularly challenging when it comes to protein sources. The thing is, that dairy, as well as legumes and all types of grains (including quinoa and whole grains), the mainstay of a vegetarian diet, are not allowed on Whole 30. And eggs are all what left for vegetarians (seafood can be the primary source of protein for pescatarians, for instance).

For the sake of the experiment, it is recommended to get all of your protein from eggs and NOT supplementing with plant-based sources (like tofu, quinoa, or Greek yogurt) for the whole month. You can take it as an excellent opportunity to evaluate how well they work for you in vegetarian life after the 30-day reset.

If you aren't up for such a sacrifice, then you'd need to modify a bit your Whole 30 to ensure your food intake is balanced and wholesome.

Here's what you get to swap in for all the meat if you are a vegetarian:

Limited dairy like yogurt and kefir

Tempeh and tofu

Whey protein powder

Hemp or pea protein powders

The thing is that after these modifications, technically, it won't be the Whole 30 reset.

List of allowed and prohibited products

What you cannot eat	What you can eat
⊖ **Sugar and any of its substitutes**, including "useful natural" one, for example, honey or stevia leaf. Instead of vanilla extract, use vanilla bean powder	✔**Eggs**
⊖**Cereals and everything that is made of cereals.** Wheat, oats, rice, and also corn are forbidden in any form, including whole grains	✔**Fruits.** Even dried fruits are allowed, although fresh ones are preferable.
⊖**All legumes, except the green beans and most peas** (such as snow peas, green peas, yellow peas, and split peas). **Strictly prohibited soybean** and all products in which it may be present.	✔**Fruit juice.** You may use it sometimes as a natural sweetener.
⊖ **Dairy products**, including fermented ones, such as yogurt or kefir. And also cheese. (Ghee or clarified butter are the only sources of dairy allowed.)	✔ **Any varieties of vegetables.** Potatoes appeared on this list in 2013.
⊖ **Any flavoring additives, flavors, preservatives** (except	✔**Nuts and seeds**, except for peanuts

balsamic, apple cider, and rice vinegar)	
⊖ **Harmful vegetable oils** - corn, sunflower, soybean oils, etc.	✓ **Useful vegetable oils** – olive oil, coconut oil
⊖ **All industrially produced food,** as there is at least one forbidden component in each of them	✓ **Coconut aminos** (it's a brewed and naturally fermented soy sauce substitute) are acceptable.

The Whole Food shopping list

I remind you that all foods should be natural (organic is not a must, but the best option). Avoid factory-made products as they usually contain harmful substances such as MSG, sulfites, or added sugar.

PROTEIN:

- Eggs

VEGETABLES:

- Acorn squash
- Artichoke
- Arugula
- Asparagus
- Beets
- Broccoli
- Bell peppers
- Brussels sprouts
- Butternut squash
- Cabbage
- Carrots

- Cauliflower
- Celery
- Cucumber
- Eggplant
- Fennel
- Garlic
- Green beans
- Jalapeno peppers
- Kale
- Leeks
- Lettuce
- Mushrooms
- Onion
- Pumpkin
- Radish
- Potatoes (all)
- Spinach
- Shallots
- Snow peas
- Spaghetti squash
- Sprouts
- Sweet Potato/Yams
- Tomato
- Turnip
- Zucchini

FRUITS:

- Apples
- Apricots
- Bananas
- Blackberries
- Blueberries
- Cherries
- Dates **
- Figs**
- Grapefruit
- Grapes
- Kiwi
- Lemon
- Lime
- Mango
- Melon
- Nectarines
- Oranges
- Papaya
- Peaches
- Plums
- Pears
- Pineapple
- Plantains
- Pomegranate

- Raspberries
- Strawberries
- Watermelon

OIL AND DRESSING:

- Coconut Oil
- Ghee
- Extra virgin olive oil
- Clarified butter
- Palm oil
- Avocado oil
- Sesame Oil

NUTS AND SEEDS:

- Cashew
- Hazelnuts
- Almonds
- Pistachio
- Walnuts
- Macadamia nuts
- Pecans
- Flax seeds
- Sesame seeds
- Sunflower seeds

HERBS AND SPICES (BOTH FRESH AND DRIED):

- Basil
- Bay leaves

- Black pepper
- Black peppercorns
- Cayenne
- Chili powder
- Chives
- Cilantro
- Cinnamon
- Cloves
- Cumin
- Curry powder
- Dill
- Garlic powder
- Ginger
- Lemongrass
- Mustard powder
- Nutmeg
- Oregano
- Paprika
- Parsley
- Red pepper flakes
- Rosemary
- Salt (sea/iodized)
- Thyme

PANTRY:

- Almond flour

- Arrowroot powder
- Apple cider vinegar*
- Balsamic vinegar*
- Cocoa (100%)
- Coconut aminos
- Coconut flour
- Dried fruits**
- Mustard*
- Raisins
- Red wine Vinegar*
- Rice vinegar*
- Tapioca starch
- Tomato paste*
- Tomatoes (dried)*
- Vegetable broth
- White vinegar*
- Olives
- Coconut/Almond milk
- Tahini
- Curry paste*
- Chili sauce*

DRINKS:

- Apple Cider
- Cacao
- Coconut water

- Coffee
- Fruit Juice
- Kombucha
- Mineral water
- Sparkling water
- Tea
- Vegetable juice

Check the labels carefully for added sugar

Limit consuming of dried fruits

The golden rules of the diet

Since Whole 30 is not just a diet for losing weight, but a way to switch to a healthy lifestyle, it has several essential rules which are strictly obligatory. If you cannot follow them all; then, do not start the program. If you break even just one of them during the clearance, you should start your Whole 30-day challenge from the beginning.

FIVE WHOLE 30 RULES
No any kind of alcohol – even as an additive to food
No smoking – during the whole month
No measuring. You are prohibited from weighing or doing any other measurements of your body during the diet. Weigh and measure the waist size on the first day of the program and then at the last one. But not in the middle of the diet
No calories counting. (However, we included the NUTRITIONal information in case you want to use these vegetarian recipes for

> ✋ **Three meals a day** is an ideal option, although dried fruits and nuts as snacks are not prohibited. But in reasonable quantities! Also, check my fabulous collection of snacks and appetizer recipes.

Also, a crucial thing to remember when doing Whole 30 clearance is to check the label on each product you purchase meticulously. A lot of prepackaged goods have added sugar or additives that you might not be aware of. We are talking about, say, mayonnaise, vinegar, tomato sauce, mustard, etc. The levels of sodium, sugar, and additives that have names you cannot even pronounce could be preventing you from maintaining a healthy weight. Becoming conscious about every bite you put in your mouth can help you achieve the healthy weight you desire and stay that way.

Whole Food expected benefits

As you have already found out, the Whole 30 cuts out potential food sensitivities for one month, as well as radically decreases inflammatory food intake and increases essential anti-inflammatory foods like veggies, fruits, and omega-3 fatty acids. Whether you have an unidentified food sensitivity or not, the overall effect of eating this way eases inflammation - so you could see subtle health improvements related to digestion, headaches, skin, and joint pain.

What else?

📌 **Weight loss: Whole 30 will help you to trim down that pesky body fat and give you an excellent body image and attractive physique**

15

✦ You won't be facing any digestive problems such as stomach bloating, farts, or tummy rumblings

✦ Improving energy potential and physical endurance

✦ Sleep normalization

✦ Giving up eating unhealthy snacks

✦ Normalization of the blood sugar and insulin levels

✦ Gaining self-confidence

✦ Reduced occurrences of depression; you will be at peace, and your anxiety levels will significantly lower down

✦ The condition of your skin will vastly improve since you are going for more vegetables and protein while eliminating sugar altogether

✦ Your hair will be healthier and shinier

✦ Workout sessions will be more productive

Thirty days of diet allow losing at least 13-15 lb of weight. Why does it happen? Because the diet eliminates processed foods that are often very high in calories derived from added sugar and fat. Eating highly processed and high-calorie foods can quickly make you gain weight, mainly because such foods lack fiber and are rich in simple sugars, which the body breaks down very fast, thus leaving you craving for more after a short period. The high-calorie content, coupled with the fact that such foods are digested quickly, means that you are likely to eat more of these, which in turn means that you will probably end up with a calorie surplus, thus increasing your chances of gaining weight.

Whole 30 foods are satiating due to their dietary fiber, which means that they take a lot of time before they can be eliminated from the body or before the body can signal you to take more food. Besides, they are rich in complex carbohydrates, which are also broken down slowly, so the likelihood of overeating such foods is small. And as such, it is easy to limit your calorie consumption even if you are not counting calories, especially because you end up eating less. The Whole 30 foods diet plan does not require any calorie counting, supplements, or complicated meal plans because it is pretty much straight forward; all you have to do is to restrict your intake of processed foods and then start eating mainly whole foods or those that are close to their natural state as possible.

The diet also improves digestion, allows normalizing carbohydrate metabolism, and is even able to help with food allergies. The Whole 30 program includes almost all groups of foods needed for adequate nutrition. The products of chemical origin (glutamates, amplifiers, and other chemical additives) are excluded from the menu, which also positively affects the state of health.

Besides, it can help a person change his/her food habits and taste preferences. Fans of the Whole 30-day diet system assure that the program does not just change eating habits, but significantly affects a person's worldview, an attitude to himself/herself, health, and lifestyle.

The Whole Food main difficulties

Doing 30 days of the whole food diet is not as hard as it seems, but it certainly requires a lot of planning. What else you have to be aware of before accepting the Whole 30 challenge?

•Social pressure

If you do not leave alone, get ready to be under the special control of your parents/beloved ones/flatmates. The first week you are going to be attacked with the questions about the diet and be at the center of family jokes – "Gosh, even no cheese?", "It's a hunger strike, not a diet," "You refused even from chewing gums? Crazy!" and so on. Everyone around will try to feed you. Be strong. And if you have the opportunity to join the program a couple more friends – do it!

•Food restrictions

Among the other foods, the diet excludes the use of milk products (except melted butter), which can negatively affect the work of the intestines, the condition of the skin, hair, and nails. For this reason, this Whole Food 30-day challenge is not recommended for pregnant and lactating women, children, and adolescent girls.

•Planning

You need to think in advance (a week or so) about what you will be eating this month. Whole 30 is not the kind of diet you can go on tomorrow. The preparation – such as doing proper shopping and creating a meal plan is required. Also, this diet on a trip or during some special occasions in your life (like your best friend's birthday) will be particularly challenging.

•Cooking

You will find it challenging to finish your whole foods diet if you do not like cooking. You have to be stuck behind the stove at least twice a day. Even people who love cooking after two weeks of the diet can get treacherous thoughts about "flakes with milk" for dinner. Stay strong! And keep reading the cookbook – my recipes are very easy to make.

Side effects of the Whole Food diet

If you have experimented with some different diets before joining the Whole 30 tribe, then you have most probably seen that there are at least "some" side effects accompanying them.

You might be wondering if the diet also has some hidden side effects as well. The good news is that you won't be facing any severe side effects. However, there have been reports of some temporary symptoms which are typical for newcomers.

Because of the total sugar elimination, you might experience mood swings, energy fluctuations, sleepiness, and food cravings. The first one-two weeks are usually the toughest. You might experience "carb flu" - you will feel sluggish while your body tries to figure out how to perform without sugar. It will pass.

Fantastic tips for the beginners

With all of those out of the way, here are some tips from those who have tried the Whole 30-day diet system and want to share their experience to make your Whole 30 journey as pleasant as possible.

☑ Make up your mind, be aware of all possible difficulties and start when you are fully committed.

☑Plan, plan, and plan one more time. Carefully plan your first-week meal plan. Then go for the next ones.

☑ Keep The Whole 30 journal: write down how you feel after each meal (ideally) and resume your day in the evenings for 30 days. Honestly, if you ask around those who have tried Whole 30, you find out that diaries have been a great tool to keep them motivated.

☑ Clear out your fridge off all foods that do not match with the diet.

☑ Plan your meals beforehand and do shopping according to it. If you are busy, keep one day aside to create your meal plan for the rest of the week. Take your lunch to the office.

☑Cook not something you should cook, but something that will make you happy and keep entertained throughout the month.

☑ Have emergency snacks in your bag, car, office, parents' house. This could be some nuts or fruits.

☑ Before starting the Whole 30, check out all the coming events... Birthdays, parties... The temptation is great. So keep your food-related socializing events at a minimum.

☑ Involve your friends, family, or housemates – it is always good to go on a diet not alone.

☑ And most importantly, never give up!

Life after your Whole Food challenge

After the monthly detox program, the second chapter of your Whole 30 begins – you have to reinstate those products that were eliminated from the diet slowly. Each group of products must be entered separately from the other. You can start with any, but the best is to choose dairy and milk products.

So, on the first day after your one-month diet has finished, you start eating dairy products. You eat them throughout the day, and then for four days, you again go back to the Whole 30 diet. It is time to watch your condition carefully.

CHAPTER 2. ONE-WEEK VEGETARIAN MEAL PLAN

To make your 30 days of the Whole Food challenge easier, we prepared this 7-day meal plan. These recipes are easy and simple to make and are great for meal prepping so that you never are caught unprepared. The best way to succeed with the Whole 30 is to plan, and we have done all the planning for you.

MONDAY	
BREAKFAST	Scrambled Eggs with Lazy Salsa
SNACK	Savory Stuffed Dates
LUNCH	Mushrooms Green Beans with Cauliflower Puree
DINNER	Roasted Veggie Salad
TUESDAY	
BREAKFAST	Apple Nut Porridge
SNACK	Flaxseed crackers
LUNCH	Hot Egg with Squash Soufflé
DINNER	Green Peas Bolognese with Pumpkin Spaghetti
WEDNESDAY	
BREAKFAST	Special Whole 30 Shakshuka
SNACK	Simple and Healthy Spinach Chips
LUNCH	Almond Pumpkin Porridge
DINNER	Special Zucchini Hummus with Garlic Sweet Potato Wedges
THURSDAY	
BREAKFAST	Super Quick Healthy Breakfast Salad

SNACK	Broccoli "Cheese" Sticks
LUNCH	Spicy Eggplant Potato Curry
DINNER	Whole Spicy No-Bean Chill
FRIDAY	
BREAKFAST	Pure Banana Chia Pudding
SNACK	Egg and Cucumber Snack
LUNCH	Whole 30 Cauliflower Tabouleh
DINNER	Baked Potato with Avocado Paste
SATURDAY	
BREAKFAST	Eggs in a Sweet Potato Nest
SNACK	Fried Eggplant Medallions
LUNCH	Spinach with Avocado "Zoodles"
DINNER	Cauliflower Falafel with Tahini Dressing and Greens
SUNDAY	
BREAKFAST	Grain-Free Apple "Oatmeal"
SNACK	Fried Plantains with Mango Salsa
LUNCH	Healthy Whole 30 Ratatouille
DINNER	Potato Cream Soup with Mushrooms

CHAPTER 3 BREAKFAST RECIPES

Simple Zucchini Noodles Bowl

Prep. time: 10 min. Cooking time: 15 min. Servings: 2

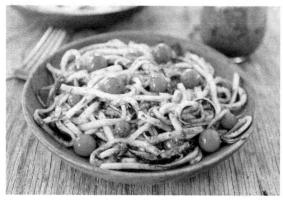

INGREDIENTS:

1 big zucchini

2 tablespoons water

¼ cup extra virgin olive oil

½ avocado

2 eggs

2 tablespoons green onions, chopped

1 garlic clove, chopped

2 sweet potatoes, peeled and cut

½ lemon (juice)

Salt and black pepper to the taste

INSTRUCTIONS:

1.Cut zucchini with the spiralizer, put aside.

2. Heat up a pan with two tablespoons of olive oil over medium-high heat, add potatoes, occasionally stir and cook for 7-8 minutes.

3. In your food processor, mix avocado with two tablespoons olive oil, garlic, water, salt, and pepper and blend well. After add a bit of lemon juice.

4. Put zucchini noodles in a bowl, add avocado cream and sweet potatoes and toss.

5. Heat up the pan where you've cooked the potatoes over medium-high heat and cook the eggs until they are done. After, transfer them to the zucchini noodles mix.

6. Add more salt and pepper, sprinkle green onions and serve.

NUTRITION:

calories 93fat 3 gfiber 3 gcarbs 11 gprotein 14 g

Apple Nut Porridge

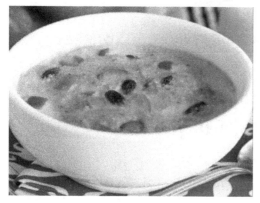

INGREDIENTS:

1/2 cup whole raw almonds

1/2 cup whole raw cashews

1/4 cup raw walnuts

1/3 cup unsweetened coconut flakes

1 large banana (should be ripe)

1 tablespoon ghee (or coconut oil)

1 apple, chopped into bite-sized pieces

1/8 teaspoon ground nutmeg

3/4 cup pure coconut milk

2 teaspoons pure vanilla extract

2 teaspoons ground cinnamon

1/2 cup raisins

Salt to the taste

Splash of almond milk (or any of your favorites)

INSTRUCTIONS:

1. In a bowl, add the nuts and coconut flakes. Pour water to cover them completely. Add salt, and cover the bowl. The nuts have to soak at least 7-8 hours or overnight. Once it's done, drain them in a colander until the water runs clear.

2. Put the nuts and coconut flakes into the food processor. Then, add a banana (break it in pieces and add to the top of the nuts). Pulse all together until it is a fine nut meal (note – not a paste).

3. Add the nutmeg and apple into the pan preheated with ghee or coconut oil. Saute the apples until they begin to get softer.

4. Add the coconut milk, cinnamon, vanilla, and raisins. After, add the banana-nut meal mixture. Stir well to mix everything.

5. Bring the porridge to a simmer and cook for 5-7 minutes until it's creamy.

6. Divide the porridge between bowls. You can add a splash of your favorite milk. Enjoy!

NUTRITION:

calories 180fat6gfiber 5,5gcarbs 24gprotein 14g

Eggs in a Sweet Potato Nest

Prep. time: 10 min. Cooking time: 25 min. Servings: 5

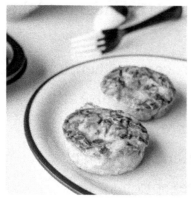

INGREDIENTS:

1 large sweet potato

1 sweet apple

2.5 tablespoons coconut oil

5 large eggs

Salt to taste

Balsamic vinegar (optional)

1 tablespoon chives (optional)

INSTRUCTIONS:

1. Preheat your oven to 350°F. Grease five cups of a jumbo muffin tin with the coconut oil. Set aside.

2. Peel the apple and potato and cut into large pieces. Then shred the apple and potato into the bowl of your food processor with the shredder attachment.

3. In a large pan, heat two tablespoons of coconut oil over medium heat. Add the shredded potato/apple and sauté until softened, or about 5 minutes, stirring occasionally. Salt to taste while cooking.

4. Scoop the potatoes out of the pan and transfer into the greased muffin cups – it is going to be around 5 cups depending on the size of your potato. Using a small cup, press an indentation into the potatoes, creating a little well in the middle and pushing the potatoes up the sides of the muffin cup. This is how you make the nest.

5. Take one egg and crack it into the center of each potato nest. Sprinkle with chives and balsamic vinegar (optional), add salt to taste. Place in the preheated oven and bake for 18-20 minutes.

6. Serve hot.

NUTRITION:

calories 205fat 14g fiber 1gcarbs 10gprotein 7g

Grain-Free Apple "Oatmeal"

Prep. time: 5 min. Cooking time: 5 min. Servings: 1

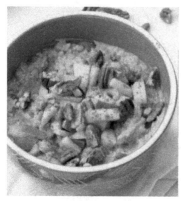

INGREDIENTS:

1/2 apple

1 date

1 tablespoon chia seeds

1 tablespoon unsweetened coconut

1 tablespoon almonds

almond butter for the topping

splash of cashew milk

INSTRUCTIONS:

1. Chop your apple and date into small (not very tiny) pieces. Then, place them in a food processor. Add the chia seeds, coconut, and almonds.

2. Pulse mixture until it's grainy and oatmeal-like. Put it in a bowl, top with milk and almond butter, and serve!

NUTRITION:

calories 79fat 5g fiber 3gcarbs 16gprotein 4g

Pure Banana Chia Pudding

Prep. time: 30 min. Cooking time: 10 min.Serving: 6 cups

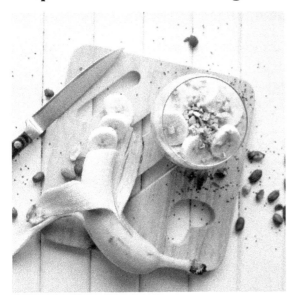

INGREDIENTS:

1 cup water

2-1/2 tablespoons chia seeds

2 ripe bananas

1 cup coconut milk

1/2 teaspoon cinnamon

Salt to the taste

Nuts for topping

INSTRUCTIONS:

1. First, let's make your chia gel. It's easy! You need to place chia seeds in a pint jar, add water and cover it. After shake it strongly and set aside for 30 minutes, occasionally shaking to break up any lumps.

2. Second, let's make your banana pudding. Combine bananas and coconut milk in a blender. Pulse until smooth. Ladle this mixture into a bowl and mix in the cinnamon, salt, and chia gel.

3. Store refrigerated and serve cold. You can top it with the nuts of your choice.

NUTRITION:

Calories 118 fat 8 g fiber 2g carbs 11g protein 1g

Scrambled Eggs with Lazy Salsa Sauce

Prep. time: 10 min.Cooking time: at least 30 min for Salsa sauce. Once it is done, egg cooking takes 5 min. Servings: 10 to 12

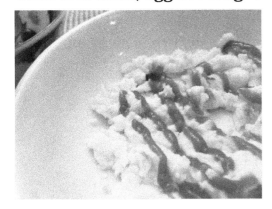

INGREDIENTS:

3 ripe tomatoes, sliced

1 bunch green onion, cut into rounds, white and light green parts only

1/2 medium red onion, diced

1 bunch cilantro, roughly chopped

1 lime

1-2 habanero chili (depends on how hot you like it!)

2 cloves garlic

Salt to the taste

2-3 eggs

INSTRUCTIONS:

1. First, you should make your salsa sauce*. Place all the ingredients, except garlic, chili, and lime, into a bowl. After mince chili and garlic, so they are almost paste-like, add it to the bowl and stir well. Squeeze the lime on top and sprinkle with salt. Toss ingredients together. Let it chill for at least 30 minutes. You can store it in the fridge for up to 5 days.

2. Second, let's make your scrambled eggs. Preheat your pan with olive oil. Whisk 2-3 eggs (per person) and cook until scrambled. Transfer them into the plates and top with salsa sauce.

* It is a good idea to make a salsa sauce in the evening. The great news is that this sauce is also good with chips, tacos, or any other meal – it depends on how much you love salsa.

NUTRITION:

Cal176 fat 7g fiber 3gcarbs 17g protein 25

Delicious Zucchini Banana Breakfast

Prep. time: 10 min. Cooking time: 10 min. Servings: 1

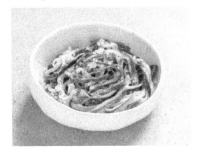

INGREDIENTS:

¾ cup vanilla almond milk

¾ cup egg whites

1 and ½ tablespoons flax seeds, ground

One small zucchini, finely grated

One small ripe banana, peeled and mashed

½ teaspoon cinnamon powder

INSTRUCTIONS:

1. Grate zucchini. Put it in a bowl, add mashed banana, stir and leave aside.

2. Heat a pan over medium heat, add milk and egg whites and mix well.

3. Add flax seeds, stir and cook for 2-3 minutes.

4. Add zucchini mix, stir and cook until the mixture thickens a bit. After, add cinnamon, stir, reduce heat to low, and cook for three more minutes.

5. Transfer to a bowl and serve right away.

NUTRITION:

calories 100fat 1gfiber 2gcarbs 0.6gprotein 4g

Super Quick Healthy Breakfast Salad

Prep. time: 5 min. Cooking time: 0 min. Servings: 1

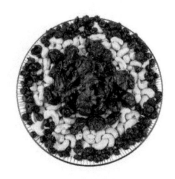

INGREDIENTS:

¼ cup raw cashews

¼ cup blueberries or raspberries (dried or fresh)

1 banana

1 tablespoon almond butter

Cinnamon powder

Coconut flakes

INSTRUCTIONS:

1. Peel and slice bananas. Then, put it in a bowl, mix with cashews and blueberries (or raspberries) and toss.

2. Add cinnamon, a pinch of coconut flakes, and almond butter, stir gently, and serve right away.

NUTRITION:

calories 90fat 0.3gfiber 1gcarbs 0gprotein 5g

Special Whole Shakshuka

Prep. time: 10 min. Cooking time: 30 min. Servings: 4

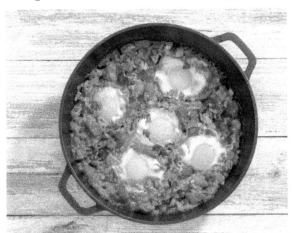

INGREDIENTS:

2 cups Brussels sprouts, chopped

1 small yellow onion, chopped

2 tablespoons extra virgin olive oil

1 middle zucchini, grated

1 teaspoon cumin

4 garlic cloves, minced

2 cups baby spinach

1 tablespoon tomato sauce

2 large tomatoes, chopped

¼ cup cilantro, chopped

4 eggs

1 avocado, pitted and sliced

Salt and black pepper to the taste

INSTRUCTIONS:

1. Heat up a pan with the oil over medium heat, add onion, stir and cook for 5 minutes. After, add garlic, stir and cook for 1 minute.

2. Add Brussels sprouts, stir and cook for another 5 minutes.

3. Add salt, pepper, cumin, cilantro, and zucchini, stir and cook for 1 minute more.

4. Add tomatoes and stir well. Then add tomato sauce.

5. Add spinach, stir, spread mix, crack eggs on top, introduce everything in the oven and cook at 375F for 7-8 minutes.

6. Garnish with avocado slices and serve hot.

NUTRITION:

calories 160fat 6g fiber 2gcarbs 9g protein 2g

Easy Baked Eggs

Prep. time: 10 min. Cooking time: 25 min. Servings: 4

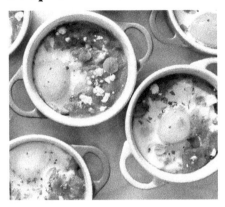

INGREDIENTS:

1 cup water

4 eggs

1 cup marinara sauce

Salt and black pepper to the taste

INSTRUCTIONS:

1. Heat up a pan with the water over medium-high heat, bring to a simmer, take off the heat and pour into a baking dish.

2. Divide marinara sauce in 4 ramekins, crack one egg in each, place ramekins in the baking dish, introduce in the oven, and cook at 350 degrees F for 25 minutes.

3. Season baked eggs with salt and pepper and serve hot.

NUTRITION:

calories 126 fat 1g fiber 0.7gcarbs 4g protein 6g

CHAPTER 4 LUNCH RECIPES

Sweet Potato and Almonds Bowl

Prep. time: 10 min. Cooking time: 10 min. Servings: 3

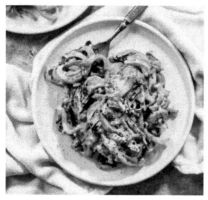

INGREDIENTS:

2 teaspoons olive oil

1 sweet potato, cut with a spiralizer

3 tablespoons almonds, sliced

1 apple, chopped with a spiralizer

3 cups spinach,

3 tablespoons raisins

Salt and pepper

For the vinaigrette:

1 teaspoon apple cider vinegar

2 tablespoons apple juice

1 tablespoon almond butter

½ teaspoon ginger, minced

1 and ½ teaspoons mustard

1 tablespoon olive oil

Salt and pepper

INSTRUCTIONS:

1. Spread almonds in a pan, introduce in the oven at 350 degrees F, and cook for 10 minutes.

2. Heat up a pan with two teaspoons of olive oil, add sweet potato noodles, stir and cook for 5 minutes.

3. Transfer potato noodles to a bowl; add salt, pepper, apple, toasted almonds, spinach, and raisins, and stir.

4. In a heatproof bowl, mix apple juice with cider vinegar and almond butter and stir.

5. Heat up in your microwave for 30 seconds and then mix with one tablespoon olive oil, ginger, salt, and mustard.

6. Whisk this well and add over potato noodles mix. Toss to coat and serve.

NUTRITION:

calories 190 fat 2g fiber 3gcarbs 7g protein 8

Whole Cauliflower Tabouleh

Prep. time: 10 min. Cooking time: 2 hours Servings: 4

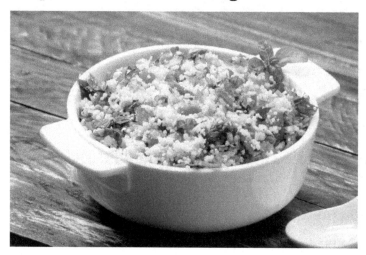

INGREDIENTS:

1/3 cup veggie stock

2 tablespoons olive oil

6 cups cauliflower florets, grated

¼ cup red onion, chopped

1 red bell pepper, chopped

½ cup kalamata olives, pitted and cut in halves

1 teaspoon mint, chopped

1 tablespoon parsley, chopped

½ lemon (juice)

Salt and pepper

INSTRUCTIONS:

1. Heat up a pan with the olive oil, add grated cauliflower, salt, pepper, and veggies, stir and cook until cauliflower is tender.

2. Transfer cauliflower rice to a bowl and keep in the fridge for 2 hours.

3. Mix cauliflower with olives, onion, bell pepper, salt, pepper, mint, parsley, and lemon juice and toss to coat.

4. Serve right away.

NUTRITION:

calories 175 fat 12g fiber 6g carbs 10gprotein 6g

Orange-Avocado Salad

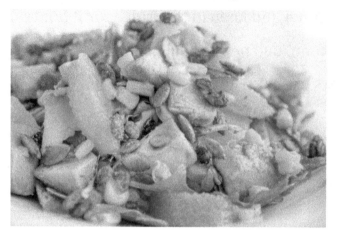

INGREDIENTS:

1 orange, cut into segments

2 green onions, chopped

1 romaine lettuce head, cut

1 avocado, pitted, peeled and chopped

¼ cup almonds, roasted and sliced

For the salad dressing:

1 teaspoon mustard

¼ cup olive oil

2 tablespoons balsamic vinegar

½ orange (juice)

Herbs (chives, dill, basil, cilantro), finely chopped

Salt and black pepper

INSTRUCTIONS:

1. In a salad bowl, mix oranges with avocado, lettuce, almonds, and green onions.

2. In a small bowl, combine olive oil with vinegar, mustard, orange juice, salt, and pepper and whisk well.

3. Add this to salad, after add herbs, mix and serve right away.

NUTRITION:

calories100fat 0.2gfiber 2gcarbs 0.4gprotein 4g

Almond Pumpkin Porridge

Prep. time: 10 min. Cooking time: 10 min. Serving: 1

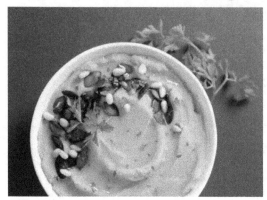

INGREDIENTS:

1 cup homemade pumpkin puree (or canned pumpkin)

⅓ cup almond pulp (leftover from making almond milk)

1 tablespoon ground flax or chia seeds

⅓ cup almond milk

½ teaspoon ground cinnamon

Toppings: nuts, dried fruit, cacao nibs

Salt to the taste

INSTRUCTIONS:

1. In a small pan, place the pumpkin, almond pulp, salt, chia or flax seeds, cinnamon, and almond milk. Whisk them together and cook until they are starting to bubble.

2. Stir the porridge for several minutes. Remove from the heat. Top with nuts or any toppings of your choice. Enjoy!

NUTRITION:

Cal 268 fat 35g fiber 10gcarbs 17g protein 16g

Sweet Potatoes Bowl

Prep. time: 10 min. Cooking time: 1 hour 15 min. Servings: 1

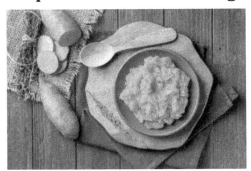

INGREDIENTS:

2 pounds sweet potatoes

2 tablespoons water

½ pound apples, cored and chopped

1 tablespoon ghee

Salt to the taste

INSTRUCTIONS:

1. Put potatoes on a lined baking sheet, introduce in the oven at 400 degrees F and bake for 1 hour.

2. Take potatoes out of the oven, leave them to cool down a bit, peel and mash them in your food processor.

3. Put apples in a pot, add the water, bring to a boil over medium heat, reduce temperature, and cook until they are soft.

4. Add this to mashed sweet potatoes, blend again, transfer to a bowl, and serve hot.

NUTRITION:

calories 80fat 1g fiber 0gcarbs 0gprotein 6g

Hot Egg with Squash Soufflé

Prep. time: 10 min. Cooking time: 1 hour Servings: 4

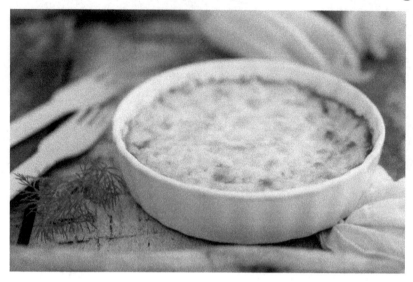

INGREDIENTS:

1 butternut squash

4 egg whites

4 egg yolks

½ cup coconut milk

Salt and black pepper to the taste

INSTRUCTIONS:

1. Bake squash in the oven at 350 degrees F for 20 minutes. After take the squash out, leave aside to cool down and scoop the flesh into the blender.

2. Add salt, pepper, egg yolks, and coconut milk and blend well.

3. In a bowl, beat egg whites.

4. Transfer squash mixture into a bowl, add egg whites, and stir.

5. Transfer this to a greased baking dish, and bake in the oven at 350 degrees F for 40 minutes.

6. Serve hot as a side dish.

NUTRITION:

calories 203fat 13g fiber 2g carbs 16g protein 4g

Spinach with Avocado "Zoodles"

Prep. time: 10 min. Cooking time: 5 min. Servings: 4

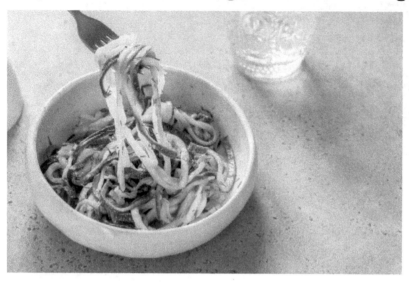

INGREDIENTS:

3 zucchinis, cut with a spiralizer

1 cup fresh basil, chopped

½ tablespoon olive oil

1 cup spinach, finely chopped

2 garlic cloves, minced

1 avocado, pitted and peeled

1/3 cup cashews, roasted

1 lemon (juice and zest)

Salt and pepper

INSTRUCTIONS:

1. Put spinach with basil, avocado, cashews, salt, lemon zest, and lemon juice in the food processor, and blend well.

2. Heat up a pan with the oil over medium-high heat, add zucchini noodles (I call them zoodles), stir, and cook for 5 minutes.

3. Add spinach and avocado sauce, stir, cook for 1 minute more, and transfer to plates.

NUTRITION:

Calories 200 fat 4g fiber 2g carbs 10gprotein 8,5g

Mushrooms Green Beans with Cauliflower Puree

Prep. time: 20 min. Cooking time: 30 min. Servings: 4

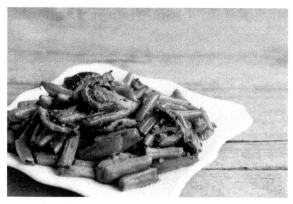

INGREDIENTS:

For cauliflower puree:

6 cups cauliflower florets

2 tablespoons ghee (or olive oil)

Salt and black pepper to the taste

For mushrooms side dish:

1 pound green beans

2 cups cremini mushrooms, chopped

1 tablespoon ghee butter

½ cup almonds, toasted and sliced

1 garlic clove, minced

Salt and black pepper to the taste

INSTRUCTIONS:

1. First, let's make our cauliflower mash. Boil water in a pot, add some salt, add cauliflower and cook for 15 minutes. Then drain and reserve 1 cup of cooking liquid.

2. In your blender, mix cauliflower with the reserved cooking liquid, salt, and pepper and blend well. Add ghee (or olive oil), mix again, and set aside.

3. Now, let's cook your mushrooms dish. Heat up a pan with the ghee butter over medium-high heat, add the garlic clove, stir and cook for 1 minute. Add mushrooms, cook for ten more minutes.

4. Add green beans, salt, and pepper, stir together and cook for 10 minutes.

5. Add almonds, stir, and take off the heat.

6. Serve the cauliflower on the plates and top it with a decent amount of the mushrooms-beans mixture.

NUTRITION:

calories 231fat 6g fiber 9gcarbs 20g protein 10g

Spicy Eggplant Potato Curry

Prep. time: 7 min. Cooking time: 25 min. Servings: 5

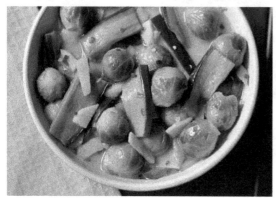

INGREDIENTS:

2 medium eggplants

1 pound brussels sprouts

5 garlic cloves, finely chopped

1 big white potato, peeled and cubed

1 can coconut milk

2 eggs, boiled and peeled

Spices: 2 tsp. turmeric, 1 tsp. dry mustard, 1/4 tsp. red pepper, 1 3/4 tsp. salt, 1 small piece ginger (finely grated)

3/4 tbsp. apple cider vinegar

3 tbsp. olive oil

1 cup water

Chopped cilantro for topping

INSTRUCTIONS:

1. Slice the eggplant lengthwise, then cut each slice into four pieces.

2. In a large skillet, add olive oil. Then, add in garlic and cook for 30 seconds over medium heat.

3. After that, add spices such as dry mustard, red pepper, turmeric, and ginger. Then stir.

4. Add eggplants, stir again, and cook for 2-3 minutes.

5. Add water, coconut milk, potato cubes, Brussels sprouts, and salt. Pour in vinegar and mix everything well.

6. Cut boiled eggs in quarters and add to the veggies.

7. Bring the curry to a boil and simmer for 15 minutes.

8. Serve hot. Top each bowl with the chopped cilantro.

NUTRITION:

calories 255fat 11.5g fiber 10.5g carbs 26g protein 7.2g

Healthy Whole Ratatouille

Prep. time: 15 min. Cooking time: 35 min. Servings: 8

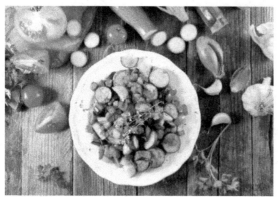

INGREDIENTS:

1 medium eggplant, cubed

1 large yellow onion, diced

2 bell peppers, seeded and chopped

2 medium zucchini, cubed

3 baby yellow squash, cubed

1/2 cup button mushrooms, sliced

1 can diced tomatoes, drained

1/3 cup tomato sauce

6 tbsp. olive oil

5 garlic cloves, minced or chopped

Spices: 1/4 tsp. crushed red pepper, 1/2 tsp. of dried thyme

Fresh greens: chopped, fresh basil, dill, and parsley to taste

Salt and pepper to taste

INSTRUCTIONS:

1. In a large pot, heat 2 tbsp. of olive oil over medium heat. Add eggplants and onions and stir well. Sprinkle with salt and pepper. Add garlic and cook for 5-7 minutes until eggplant is brown. Set aside in a bowl.

2. In the same pot, add mushrooms and red pepper and cook for about 2-3 minutes. Add them in the bowl with eggplant.

3. Add 2 tbsp. of olive oil In the same pot. Place in bell peppers, cubed zucchini, and baby yellow squash. Sauté for 3-4 minutes.

4. Add in the pot eggplant/mushrooms mixture.Then add diced tomatoes, tomato sauce, and thyme. Stir well and bring to a boil. Lower heat and simmer for about 17-20 minutes.

5. Before serving, top with basil, dill, and parsley. It also tastes cold!

NUTRITION:

calories 271 fat 9.3g fiber 8.4g carbs 27g protein 9.2g

CHAPTER 5 SAUCE RECIPES

Whole Salsa Sauce

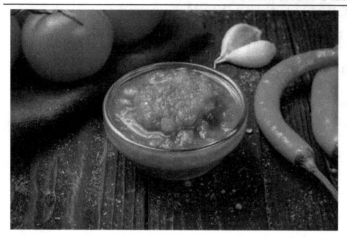

INGREDIENTS:

3 ripe tomatoes, sliced

1 bunch green onion, sliced

1/2 medium red onion, diced

1 bunch cilantro, roughly chopped

1 lime

1-2 habanero chili (depends on how hot you like it!)

2 cloves garlic

Salt to taste

INSTRUCTIONS:

1. Place all the ingredients, except garlic, chili, and lime, into a bowl.

2. In a separate small bowl, mince chili and garlic, so they are almost paste-like.

3. Add chili and garlic to the bowl with all the ingredients and stir well.

4. Squeeze the lime on top and sprinkle with salt.

5. Toss ingredients together. Chill for at least 30 minutes. It can be in a fridge for up to 5 days.

NOTE: It is a good idea to make a salsa sauce in the evening. It is also good with chips, tacos, or any other meal – depends on how much you love salsa.

Homemade Mayonnaise

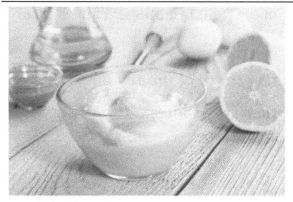

INGREDIENTS:

1/4 cup + 1 more cup of light olive oil (light, not extra virgin)

1 egg

1/2 teaspoon mustard powder (check the label for additional sugar)

1/2 teaspoon salt

1/2 to 1 lemon, juiced

INSTRUCTIONS:

1. Make sure that all ingredients (the lemon and egg) are at room temperature.

2. In a food processor (or blender), mix the egg, 1/4 cup of olive oil, mustard powder, and salt.

3. Slowly drizzle 1 cup of olive oil in the food processor while it is running. NOTE: you have to pour that olive oil as slowly as possible. The slower you pour, the thicker your mayo will be.

4. After add lemon* juice to taste, stirring gently with a spoon to incorporate.

_ NOTE: a lemon goes last._*

Delicious Worcestershire Sauce

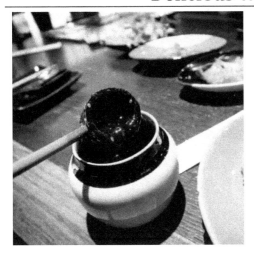

INGREDIENTS:

1/2 cup Apple Cider Vinegar

3 tbsp. date paste (ground up dates with a little water)

2 tbsp. coconut aminos

3 tbsp. water

Juice of 1 lime

1/2 tsp. dry mustard

1/4 tsp. ground ginger

1/4 tsp. onion powder

1/4 tsp. garlic powder

1/4 tsp. ground cinnamon

1/8 tsp. black pepper

1/8 tsp. cayenne pepper

INSTRUCTIONS:

1. Put all the ingredients in a medium saucepan and stir to combine over medium heat.

2. Stir constantly. Bring to a boil. Let simmer for 1-2 minute(s).

3. Remove from heat and let it cool. Store in a glass bottle in the refrigerator. It can be stored for up to 2 months.

Note: It is quite difficult to find Whole 30 compliant Worcestershire sauce in stores. It's either got soy sauce or artificial sugar in it. Your homemade Worcestershire sauce is the best choice to make sure you do not break your whole 30 challenge.

Dairy-Free Basil Pesto

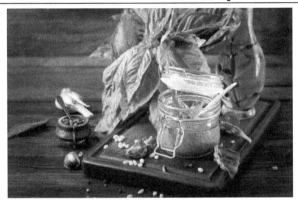

INGREDIENTS:

2 cups fresh basil

1/2 cup extra virgin olive oil

1 cup cashews raw and unsalted

3 tbsp. nutritional yeast

2 garlic cloves garlic

1/4 tsp. salt

1/4 tsp. pepper

INSTRUCTIONS:

1. Add all the listed ingredients (use just a half of olive oil and set aside the rest) to a food processor or blender. Pulse a few times.

2. Add the remaining olive oil. Turn the food processor or blender to a low speed. Blend until smooth, but before it gets creamy.

3. Season to taste with salt and pepper.

Note: Do not forget to cover the pesto. You can store it in the fridge for up to 5 days. Alternately, you can add it to ice cube trays and freeze into cubes.

Whole Marinara Sauce

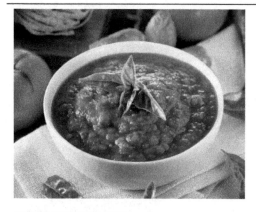

INGREDIENTS:

1 large can diced tomatoes

1 cup water

1/4 cup olive oil

7 garlic cloves, sliced

Spices: red pepper flakes, dried oregano, dried basil, and salt to taste

INSTRUCTIONS:

1. Take tomatoes out of the can and crush with your hands. Set aside the tomato juice from the can.

2. Heat up olive oil in a skillet over medium heat. Add in garlic and cook for 30 seconds or so, not allowing it to brown.

3. Add in tomatoes, and tomato juice from the can and stir well. Add in salt, red pepper flakes, basil, and oregano. Mix well.

4. Pour in a bit of water, turn the heat down to low and simmer for about 15 minutes, or until thickened. Mix thoroughly and use as needed.

CHAPTER 6 SNACKS & APPETIZERS RECIPES

Flaxseed Crackers

Prep. time: check the recipe Cooking time: 1 hour Servings: 1

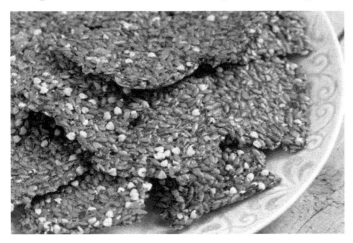

INGREDIENTS:

1 cup flaxseeds

2 cups water

½ teaspoon salt

2 teaspoons fresh rosemary, chopped

1 teaspoon lemon juice

INSTRUCTIONS:

1. You will need a medium bowl. Put in 1 cup of flaxseeds and add s of water. Mix and leave it for at least one hour or even overnight.

2. After the flaxseed mixture has set, the water in the mixture should form a gel-like consistency.

3. Line a large baking sheet with parchment paper. Add the salt, rosemary, and lemon juice, then pour a thin layer on the sheet.

4. Preheat your oven to 325 degrees and bake your crackers for an hour until crispy.

5. Once the flaxseed crackers are in consistency, simply break off the sheet into small-bite sized portions.

NUTRITION:

calories 45fat 0g fiber 1gcarbs 5g protein 0g

Fried Eggplant Medallions

Prep. time: 15 min. Cooking time: 15 min. Servings: 2

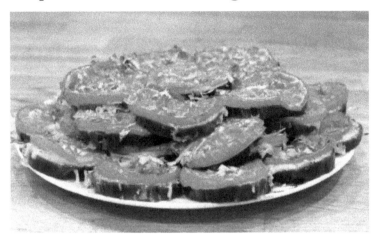

INGREDIENTS:

2 eggplants, cut into slices

2 tomatoes, cut into slices

1 garlic clove, finely minced

1 teaspoon cilantro, finely minced

1 teaspoon dill, finely minced

2 tablespoons homemade mayonnaise

1 tablespoon olive oil

Salt and pepper

INSTRUCTIONS:

1. In the bowl, put eggplants slices, add salt and pepper and stir gently. Leave for 10-15 minutes.

2. After that, heat up a pan, add olive oil, put eggplants slices in, and fry until both sides are brown.

3. Transfer on the plate to cool down.

4. In a small bowl, mix mayonnaise, garlic, cilantro, and dill. Smear eggplants slices with mayonnaise mixture.

5. Put tomato slices on top of each eggplant slices. Leave it to cool in the fridge for 30 minutes.

NUTRITION:

calories 37 fat 2g fiber 1g carbs 9g protein 0g

Egg and Cucumber Snack

Prep. time: 10 min. Cooking time: 7 min. Servings: 1

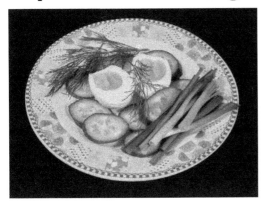

INGREDIENTS:

2 eggs

1 cucumber, cut into medium slices

1 tablespoon dill, chopped

¼ teaspoon paprika

Salt and black pepper

INSTRUCTIONS:

1. Put some water in a pot, add eggs, bring to a boil over medium heat, cook for 7 minutes, drain and transfer to a bowl filled with cold water.

2. Cool down eggs, peel them, and slice them.

3. Arrange cucumber slices on a plate, add egg slices on top, sprinkle salt, pepper, and paprika, and serve with dill on top.

NUTRITION:

calories 170fat 5g fiber 1gcarbs 2g protein 14g

Fried Plantains with Mango Salsa

Prep. time: 10 min. Cooking time: 10 min. Servings: 4

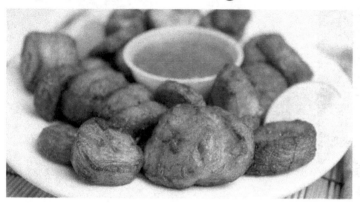

INGREDIENTS:

4 green plantains, peeled and each cut into 2-inch pieces

4 cups coconut oil

Salt

For the mango salsa:

1 avocado, pitted, peeled and cubed

2 cups mango, cubed

¼ cup cilantro, chopped

½ cup red onion, chopped

2 tablespoons olive oil

Salt and black pepper to the taste

1 lime (juice)

A pinch of red pepper flakes

INSTRUCTIONS:

1. Heat up a pan with the coconut oil over medium-high heat, add plantain pieces, fry for 5 minutes on both sides, and transfer to paper towels.

2. Place plantains on a sheet of parchment paper, add another one over them, and press with a meat pounder.

3. Heat up the pan with the oil again over medium-high heat, add plantain patties, cook them for 5 minutes more, drain on paper towels and arrange on a platter.

4. In a bowl, mix avocado with mango, onion, and cilantro.

5. Add olive oil, salt, pepper, and pepper flakes, toss to coat, and serve your plantains with the salsa on the side.

NUTRITION:

calories 200fat 3g fiber 9g carbs 8g protein 12g

Savory Stuffed Dates

Prep. time: 10 min. Cooking time: 0 min. Servings: 1

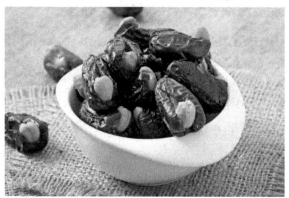

INGREDIENTS:

2 Medjool dates, cut on one side

5 pistachios, raw and chopped

1 teaspoon coconut, shredded

INSTRUCTIONS:

1. In a bowl, mix chopped pistachios with coconut and stir very well.

2. Stuff each date with this mix and serve them right away.

NUTRITION:

calories 60fat 1g fiber 0gcarbs 0.2g protein 1g

Marvelous Energy Snacks

Prep. time: 10 min. Cooking time: 12 min. Servings: 8

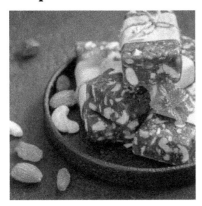

INGREDIENTS:

1 cup dried fruits

1 cup dates, pitted and dried

1 cup nuts mix (cashew, walnuts)

INSTRUCTIONS:

1. Spread nuts on a lined baking sheet and roast in the oven at 350 degrees F for 15 minutes. After nuts have cooled down, put them in the food processor.

2. Add dried fruit and dates and blend well. After, shake the processor a bit and pulse again for 2 minutes.

3. Spread this on a wax paper, press dough well into a square, cover, and keep in the fridge for 1 hour.

4. Cut into 8 bars and serve as a snack.

NUTRITION:

calories 200fat 7g fiber 4g carbs 41g protein 4g

Simple and Healthy Spinach Chips

Prep. time: 10 min. Cooking time: 10 min. Servings: 3

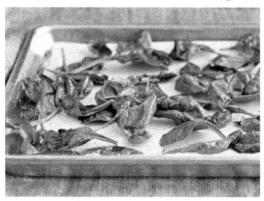

INGREDIENTS:

2 cups baby spinach

A pinch of garlic powder

½ tablespoon extra-virgin olive oil

Salt and black pepper

INSTRUCTIONS:

1. Wash and pat dry baby spinach leaves; after, spreads them on a lined baking sheet.

2. In a bowl, mix oil with salt, pepper, and garlic powder and whisk well.

3. Drizzle this over spinach, toss to coat, spread leaves again and bake in the oven at 325 degrees F for 10-12 minutes.

4. Leave spinach chips to cool down before serving.

NUTRITION:

calories 75fat 4g fiber 1.5g carbs 2.4g protein 2g

Broccoli "Cheese" Sticks

Prep. time: 20 min. Cooking time: check the recipe

Servings: 22 sticks

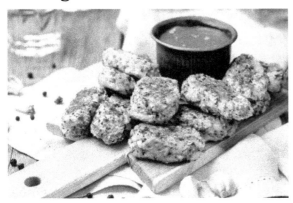

INGREDIENTS:

4 cups broccoli florets

1 cup almond flour

¼ cup coconut flour

¼ teaspoon onion powder

¼ teaspoon garlic powder

½ teaspoon salt

1 large egg

½ teaspoon apple cider vinegar (check the label for sugar additives)

INSTRUCTIONS:

1. Preheat oven to 375 degrees. After, add the broccoli florets in a pot with boiling water. Boil for 8-10 minutes, until broccoli is soft, and drain the water.

2. Add the broccoli to a food processor and pulse until it is paste-like. Transfer it into a bowl.

3. In another bowl, combine the almond flour, coconut flour, onion powder, garlic powder, and salt. Add it to the broccoli, then add the egg and vinegar and mix well.

4. Pour the mixture on a parchment-lined baking sheet and place another piece of parchment paper over the top. Using a rolling pin, spread the down by pressing it out on the top piece of parchment paper until it's roughly ⅓ - ½ inch thick.

5. Remove the top part of the parent paper. Using a pizza cutter, score the dough to make sticks.

6. Preheat your oven to 375 degrees. Bake the sticks for about 30 minutes. Let them cool.

7. Place in the fridge. You can freeze any leftover sticks and thaw when needed.

8. Serve with any sauce of your choice! (Check Chapter 6. Sauce Recipes.)
NUTRITION:

calories 110fat 3g fiber 3gcarbs 11g protein 5g

CHAPTER 7 DINNER RECIPES

Baked Potato with Avocado Paste

Prep. time: 10 min. Cooking time: 40 min. Servings: 3

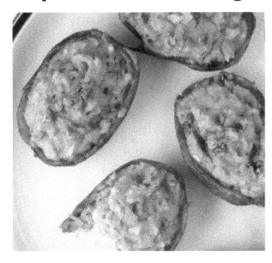

INGREDIENTS:

3 potatoes, cut into two

1 avocado, pitted and sliced

1 lime (juice)

2 tablespoons extra virgin olive oil

Garlic powder

1 tablespoon chives, chopped

1 tablespoon cilantro, chopped

1 teaspoon sesame seeds

Salt, red and black pepper to taste

INSTRUCTIONS:

1. Heat up an oven over medium-high heat, add potato slices, season with salt, pepper, garlic powder, and drizzle the oil.

2. Bake for 35-40 minutes at 375°F.

3. In the bowl, mix avocado, salt and pepper, red pepper, lime juice, sesame seeds, chives, cilantro, and stir gently.

4. Top each potato slice with avocado paste and serve.

NUTRITION:

calories 100 fat 7g fiber 1gcarbs 5g protein 10g

Green Peas Bolognese with Pumpkin Spaghetti

Prep. time: 15 min. Cooking time: 20 min. Servings: 4

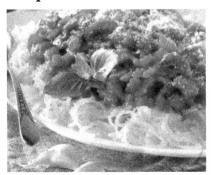

INGREDIENTS:

For peas Bolognese:

4 cups green peas (frozen)

1 yellow onion, finely chopped

2 cups vegetable broth

3 garlic cloves, finely chopped

1 tsp. nutritional yeast (make sure, it's gluten-free)

1 tsp. Homemade Worcestershire sauce (check the recipe here)

1 tbsp. balsamic vinegar

2 tbsp. ghee

1 can whole tomatoes (check the label for additives!)

1 tbsp. tomato paste (check the label for added sugar OR see how to make it here)

3 tbsp. almond flour

1 tsp.basil

1 tsp. oregano

Salt and pepper to taste

For vegetable spaghetti:

1 butternut pumpkin, peeled and cut into thin strips

1 tbsp. olive oil

A handful of baby spinach leaves

Juice from one orange

Fresh herbs

Salt and pepper to taste

INSTRUCTIONS:

1. First, let's make your peas Bolognese. Heat up a large skillet with the ghee butter and add chopped onion and garlic. Fry for 30 seconds and turn off the heat.

2. In a blender, add canned tomatoes, almond flour, basil, and oregano. Blend well.

3. Add nutritional yeast, tomato paste, Worcestershire sauce, and balsamic vinegar to the skillet and turn the heat on. Stir in tomato/herbs mixture and cook for 2-3 minutes.

4. Add vegetable broth. Cook over low heat until thickened. Finally, add the green peas, mix and sauté cook for another 3 minutes. Let it chill.

5. Now, it's time to make our orange pumpkin spaghetti. Heat up a pan with olive oil. Add pumpkin strips and sauté over medium heat for 2-3 minutes.

6. Season with orange juice, salt, and black pepper.

7. Add fresh herbs and baby spinach leaves.

8. Divide between serving plates and top with green peas Bolognese.

NUTRITION:

calories 232fat 6g fiber 3.6gcarbs 16g protein 5.9g

Ruddy Zucchini Sweet Potato Pancakes

Prep. time: 15 min. Cooking time: 10 min. Servings: 4

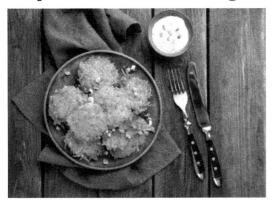

INGREDIENTS:

1 cup zucchini, grated

1 cup sweet potato, shredded

1 tablespoon coconut flour

1 egg, whisked

¼ teaspoon cumin, ground

½ teaspoon garlic powder

½ teaspoon parsley, dried

1 tablespoon extra-virgin olive oil

1 tablespoon ghee

Salt and black pepper to the taste

Herbs – chives, cilantro, dill (additional)

2 tablespoons homemade mayonnaise(see here how to make it)

INSTRUCTIONS:

1. In a bowl, mix flour with salt, pepper, cumin, garlic powder, and parsley.

2. In another bowl, combine zucchini with egg and sweet potato and stir.

3. Combine the two mixtures and stir well. Add herbs (if you want) and stir.

4. Heat up a pan with the oil and ghee over medium-high heat, shape pancakes from zucchini mix, drop them into the pan, cook until they are gold, flip and cook until they turn golden on the other side as well.

5. Transfer to paper towels, drain grease, divide between plates, top with the mayonnaise, and serve hot.

NUTRITION:

calories 122fat 8g fiber 2g carbs 7g protein 3g

Roasted Veggie Salad

Prep. time: min. 25 Cooking time: 25 min. Servings: 4

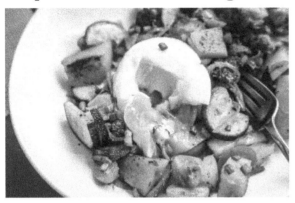

INGREDIENTS:

2 cups red potatoes, cut into small cubes

1/2 medium red bell pepper, sliced

1/2 medium yellow bell pepper, sliced

1 cup mushrooms, halved

1/2 cup zucchini, sliced

½ cup eggplant, sliced

1 tbsp. garlic, minced

1/4 cup olive oil

2 tsp. dried rosemary

1/2 tsp. black pepper

2 tsp. balsamic vinegar

1 egg, boiled

Cilantro and basil, for garnish

INSTRUCTIONS:

1. Place cubed potatoes in a large pot of water and boil for 10 minutes. Drain water, add fresh water, and cook until tender.

2. Add the bell peppers, garlic, mushrooms, zucchini, olive oil, and rosemary to the pot. Mix well. Cook for another 5 minutes. Drain water.

3. Line your broiler pan with an aluminum foil (to keep up juices and speed up cleaning) and spread your veggies on it. Season with black pepper and broil for about 15 minutes. Stir a few times during cooking.

4. Add veggies back to the large pot and toss with the balsamic vinegar. Top with chopped boiled egg.

5. Serve hot or at room temperature.

6. Garnish with cilantro or basil.

NUTRITION:

calories 220 fat 16g fiber 3gcarbs 17g protein 3g

Special Zucchini Hummus with Garlic Sweet Potato Wedges

Prep. time: 15 min. Cooking time: 50 min. Servings: 6

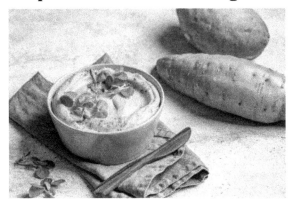

INGREDIENTS:

For zucchini hummus:

2 zucchinis, chopped

1 tablespoon coconut oil

4 garlic cloves, chopped

½ cup tahini

1 tbsp. turmeric

2 tablespoons lemon juice

4 ounces roasted peppers, chopped

Salt and black pepper to the taste

For potato wedges:

6 sweet potatoes

10 garlic cloves, minced

6 tbsp. olive oil

Salt and pepper to taste

INSTRUCTIONS:

1. First, let's make our hummus. Spread zucchinis on a baking sheet, add salt, pepper, and the oil, toss to coat, and bake in the oven at 400 degrees F for 20 minutes.

2. Take zucchinis out of the oven, leave aside to cool down for 10 minutes, and transfer to your food processor.

3. Add more salt and pepper, tahini, garlic, lemon juice, and roasted peppers and blend well. Let it chill in the fridge for an hour or so.

4. Now let's cook our sweet potatoes. Preheat oven to 425F. Halve sweet potatoes and cut each half into 1/2 inch wedges.

5. Heat olive oil in a large skillet. Add in sweet potato wedges and cook until golden brown, about 3-4 minutes per side.

6. Place sweet potatoes on a foil-lined baking sheet. Add garlic, season with salt and pepper, and toss. Roast for 10-15 minutes, then toss and roast for another 8-9 minutes.

7. Transfer the hummus into the bowl. Serve with hot sweet potato wedges.

NUTRITION:

calories 340 fat 8.9g fiber 4.3gcarbs 13g protein 9.5g

Whole Spicy No-Bean Chill

Prep. time: min. 25 Cooking time: 45 min. Servings: 6

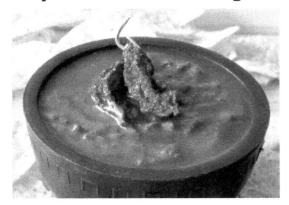

INGREDIENTS:

1 medium onion, diced

2 garlic cloves, minced

1 green bell pepper, diced

1 red bell pepper, diced

2 carrots, peeled and diced

1 medium zucchini, cut into small cubes

1 small eggplant, diced

1 banana pepper, deseeded, minced

1 jalapeño pepper, deseeded, minced

28 ounces diced tomatoes

3 cups vegetable broth (plus 3 tbsp. for sautéing)

Spices: 1 tbsp. chili powder, 2 tsp. smoked paprika, 1 tbsp. cumin,

Fresh herbs: handful oregano and cilantro, chopped (for garnish)

Salt and pepper to taste

INSTRUCTIONS:

1. Put in 3 tbsp. of vegetable broth in a big saucepan, add the diced onion and cook over medium heat for 4-5 minutes.

2. Add bell peppers, banana pepper, and jalapeño peppers and stir well.

3. Add in garlic and carrots and stirring sauté for 5 minutes. You can add in a bit of veggie broth if the vegetables start to stick.

4. Add the eggplant, zucchini, and spices, mix well, and sauté for about 2 minutes.

5. Add the diced tomatoes and veggie broth, bring to a simmer and keep cooking for about 12-15 minutes until bubbly and thick.

6. Season with salt and pepper to your taste. Simmer for another 5 minutes.

7. Serve hot garnished with fresh oregano and cilantro.

NUTRITION:

calories 178fat 1g fiber 5.8g carbs 13.9g protein 4.2g

* NOTES:

- Do not remove the seeds out of the hot peppers if you like your chili super spicy

- Do not add in both the jalapeño or banana pepper, if you like your chili less spicy

- Start with 2 cups of veggie broth. If you like it soupier, add an extra cup.

Cheesy Spinach Artichoke in Baked Potato Boats

Prep. time: 10 min. Cooking time: 1 hour 30 min. Servings: 6-8

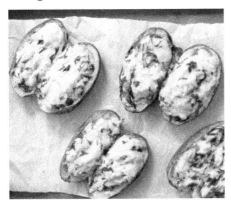

INGREDIENTS:

4 medium russet potatoes, washed

½ cup fresh baby spinach

1/2 of a 14 oz can artichoke hearts, chopped

1/2 medium yellow onion, diced

2 garlic cloves, minced

1 small can coconut cream

1.5 tbsp. fresh lemon juice

3/4 tsp. sea salt

2 tbsp. nutritional yeast

2 tbsp. ghee butter

INSTRUCTIONS:

1. Let's prepare our potato boats first. Preheat your oven at 400F. Then rub the washed potatoes with coconut oil and season with salt. Bake them for about 1 hour or until soft inside (use the toothpick to check it)*. Set aside to cool.

2. Once cooled, cut each potato open lengthwise and scoop out the inside, leaving a thin layer - so they would look like little boats. Keep the potato mash; you will need it.

3. Heat a medium skillet over medium heat and add 1 tbsp. ghee butter. Add diced onion and cook for 2-3 minutes, then add the garlic, stir well.

4. Then stir in the spinach and sautée for 1-2 minutes. Add the chopped artichoke hearts, sprinkle with salt and cook one more minute. Remove from heat and set aside.

5. In a large bowl, mix the leftover from the potatoes, coconut cream, lemon juice, ghee, nutritional yeast, and salt.

6. Combine the potato mixture with the spinach/artichoke mixture. Then, with the spoon, scoop it into the hollowed potato boats.

7. Place your stuffed potatoes in the oven and bake at 400F for about 18-20 minutes until they are lightly brown. Remove from oven and serve hot.

* NOTE: If you're short on time, bake the potatoes ahead of time and store in the refrigerator until ready to proceed with the recipe.
NUTRITION:
calories 282 fat 9.9g fiber 6.3g carbs 16g protein 6.9g

Cauliflower Falafel with Tahini Dressing and Greens

Prep. time: 10 min. Cooking time: 40 min. Servings: 8

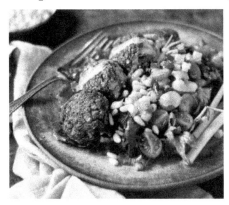

INGREDIENTS:

For falafel:

1 cup cauliflower, minced in food processor

1 large yellow onion, minced

1/4 cup fresh cilantro leaves

1/4 cup fresh parsley leaves

1/4 cup almond flour

1 egg

1/2 tbsp. arrowroot flour

2 garlic cloves

Spices: 2 tsp. cumin powder, 1/2 tsp. sea salt, 1/4 tsp. turmeric powder,

1/4 tsp. chili powder

2 tbsp. olive oil

For tahini dressing:

1/4 cup sesame oil

1/8 cup tahini

1 tbsp. lemon juice + 1/4 tsp. lemon zest

1 tsp. date paste

Greens:

2 cup baby kale, chopped

1/2 cup cherry tomatoes, cut in halves

1/8 cup pine nuts

1/8 cup fresh cilantro leaves, finely chopped

1/8 cup dill, finely chopped

INSTRUCTIONS:

1. Let`s make your falafel first. Preheat oven to 400F. Line a baking sheet with parchment paper.

2. In a food processor, place all the falafel ingredients, except the minced cauliflower and olive oil, and blend until the herbs are minced.

3. Then, add in the cauliflower and pulse until combined.

4. Make medium round balls out of the falafel dough. Brush them with olive oil (use a pastry brush).

5. Place them in the oven and bake for 20 minutes. Then rotate the falafels and cook for another 20 minutes.

6. To make the dressing, place all the tahini dressing ingredients in a blender (or food processor) and blend until smooth.

7. Serve your salads on the plates, then top with falafel and tahini dressing.

NUTRITION:

calories 180fat 20g fiber 3gcarbs 8gprotein 4g

Potato Cream Soup with Mushrooms

Prep. time: 15 min. Cooking time: 20 min. Servings: 6

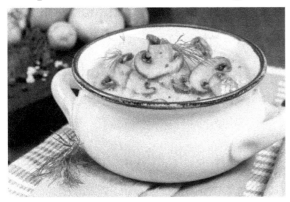

INGREDIENTS:

6-8 medium potatoes

1 cup champignon mushrooms

1 large carrot

½ tsp. dried dill

2 tbsp. olive oil

Salt to the taste

A handful of finely chopped cilantro

INSTRUCTIONS:

1. Wash, peel, and cut potatoes into the cubes (the smaller they are, the faster they will be cooked). Place them in a saucepan, pour in water, and bring to a boil.

2. Once the water has boiled, add in salt to your taste. Cook it for 10-15 min. and set aside.

3. Wash and grate carrots finely. Wash mushrooms and slice them.

4. Heat up olive oil in a medium skillet over medium heat and add in the grated carrots. Cook tossing for 2-3 minutes. Add the mushrooms. Mix well and keep cooking for 5 minutes more. Sprinkle with salt but remember that you've already added some salt to the potatoes.

5. Drain the water from the potatoes into another pot. Then mash the potatoes with the spoon, or you can use a blender. After slowly pour in the "potato water" again, continually stirring until it's thick and creamy. (Note you could need the rest of the water to add to the soup later when it is too thick.)

6. Add mushrooms in the soup. Mix. Add dried drill. Mix again. Serve hot! You can top your creamy soup with chopped cilantro if you wish.

NUTRITION:

calories 195 fat 4.9g fiber 5.5g carbs 32.1g protein 4.1g

Whole Light Beet Soup

Prep. time: 20 min. Cooking time: 20 min. Servings: 6

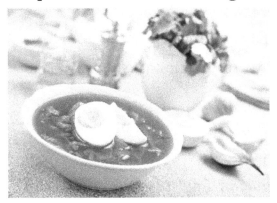

INGREDIENTS:

1 large beet, chopped into cubes or grated

1 large carrot, grated

1 medium yellow onion, finely chopped

4 medium potatoes, cut into cubes

1 tomato

1 bell pepper, cut into strips

2 tbsp. tomato paste

6 whole black peppercorns

2 bay leaf

2 tbsp. olive oil

1 egg, boiled

Greens: cilantro, dill, basil, parsley to taste

Salt to taste

INSTRUCTIONS:

1. Place potato cubes in a large saucepan, pour in water and cook over medium heat. Bring it to boil and set aside.

2. Meanwhile, let's cook the veggies. Heat up a medium skillet with olive oil. Add in beetroot cubes and fry for 1-2 minutes. Add chopped onion and grated carrots and stirring cook for 1-2 minutes.

3. Peel tomato, finely chop and add to the same skillet. Add in tomato paste and mix well. You can add a bit of water (optional). Cook for 1-2 minutes.

4. Transfer fried veggies into the saucepan and mix with potatoes. Add in bell pepper strips and chopped greens.

5. Add black peppercorns, bay leaves, and sprinkle with salt.

6. Serve it either hot or cold. Top with the boiled egg, chopped in halves.

NUTRITION:

calories 176fat 5g fiber 5.3g carbs 31g protein 3.7g

CHAPTER 8 DESSERTS RECIPES

Baked Almond Butter Banana "Boats"

Prep. time: 3 min. Cooking time: 15 min. Servings: 1

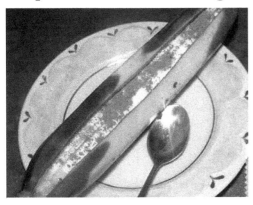

INGREDIENTS:

1 large banana

½ teaspoon cinnamon

1 tablespoon almond butter

INSTRUCTIONS:

1. Preheat your oven to 375 degrees. Cut about ½ deep down the length of the banana.

2. Widen the cut with a spoon, making a place for the almond butter.

3. Fill in with the butter. Sprinkle with cinnamon.

4. Wrap completely in foil and bake for 15 minutes.

5. Allow it to cool for a few minutes, unwrap, and serve.

NUTRITION:

Calories 206 fat 9.4gfiber 5.3g carbs 31g protein 4.7g

Five-Minute Cranberry Nuts Bites

Prep. time: 5 min. Cooking time: 5 min. Servings: 16 bites

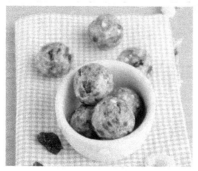

INGREDIENTS:

1 cup almonds

1 cup cashews

1 cup dates

1 cup dried cranberries 130 g

1 teaspoon vanilla bean powder

1 lemon (zest + juice)

1/4 teaspoon salt

INSTRUCTIONS:

1. In a food processor, put the cashew and almonds until coarse. Then add dates, cranberries, vanilla bean powder, lemon, and salt, and blitz until blended.

2. Roll into bite-sized balls. Place in an airtight container in the fridge for 30 minutes.

NUTRITION:

calories 125 fat 7 g fiber 2 g carbs 15 g protein 3

Coconut Berry Mix Tarts

Prep. time: 5 min. Cooking time: 5 min. Servings: 16 pieces

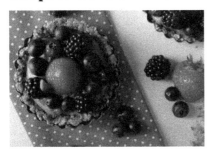

INGREDIENTS:

14 Medjool dates, pits removed

¼ cup almonds

1 can coconut milk

¼ cup raspberries

¼ cup strawberries, sliced

INSTRUCTIONS:

1. In a food processor, put almonds and dates and process for about 1 minute until there are no big chunks.

2. Line two small springform pans with parchment paper. Divide the mixture between the two pans and, with hands, press it to form a crust.

3. In a bowl, put coconut milk and whip it for a minute with a hand mixer, then add the spoonful of the mixture that you've made and five raspberries. Beat until combined.

4. Put the coconut cream into the tart crusts and then top the tarts with raspberries and strawberries.

NUTRITION:

calories 110 fat 5g fiber 1gcarbs 11gprotein 1g

Blueberry Banana Cream

Prep. time: 5 min. Cooking time: 5 min. Servings: 4

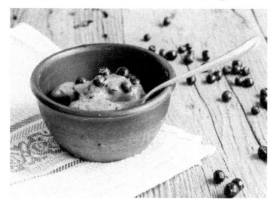

INGREDIENTS:

3 cups frozen bananas

1 cup frozen blackberries

1 tablespoon fresh mint

INSTRUCTIONS:

1. Peel and roughly chop bananas before freezing.

2. In a food processor, blend banana, blackberries, and mint until smooth and creamy. If necessary, allow bananas to thaw for a few minutes before blending. Serve immediately.

NUTRITION:

calories 90fat 0 fiber 4g carbs 22gprotein 1,5g

Mango Chia Pudding

Prep. time: 10 min. Cooking time: 10 min. Servings: 4

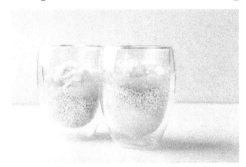

INGREDIENTS:

1 can of coconut milk

¼ cup chia seeds

2 mangos, peeled and smashed into a puree

2 limes

INSTRUCTIONS:

1. Pour the coconut milk into a large bowl and whisk thoroughly. Add in the chia seeds and stir thoroughly to combine. Leave the chia pudding in the fridge for at least 4 hours but preferably overnight.

2. Divide the mango puree into four small bowls. Two tablespoons leave aside as a topping.

3. Top all the bowls with chia pudding.

4. Grate lime zest over the tops of the pudding, then cut the lime into wedges. Squeeze a lime wedge over the chia pudding. Serve with additional sliced lime wedges.

NUTRITION:

calories 86fat 2g fiber 5g carbs 15g protein 1g

Banana Almond Brownie

Prep. time: 1 min. Cooking time: 10 min. Servings: 1

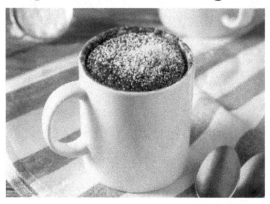

INGREDIENTS:

1 large ripe banana

1 tablespoon almond butter

1 tablespoon cocoa powder

A pinch coconut flakes

INSTRUCTIONS:

1. Mash your ripe banana, then add almond butter and cocoa powder and mix very well.

2. Grease a mug with some butter, transfer the banana mixture, and top with coconut flakes.

3. Bake in an oven for 10-12 minutes at 350 degrees until cooked.

NUTRITION:

calories 135fat 7g fiber 3gcarbs 17g protein 1.8g

Baked Cinnamon Apples with Sweet Potato

Prep. time: 1 min. Cooking time: 10 min. Servings: 1

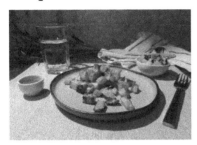

INGREDIENTS:

2 apples, sliced

2 sweet potatoes, peeled and sliced into rounds

2 tablespoon ghee

2 tablespoon water

2 teaspoon cinnamon

Salt

INSTRUCTIONS:

1. Preheat oven to 375°F.

2. In a casserole dish, put apples, potatoes, ghee, cinnamon, and water. Mix until apples and sweet potatoes are evenly coated. Cover with foil and place in the oven for 30 minutes.

3. Remove foil, stir and bake for 15-20 minutes more tossing again halfway through baking time.

4. Remove from oven, sprinkle with a little salt and serve.

NUTRITION:

calories 140 fat 5g fiber 3.8g carbs 22g protein 1g

Fruit Popsicles

Prep. time: 1 min. Cooking time: 10 min. Servings: 1-3

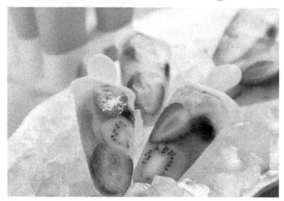

INGREDIENTS:

Coconut water

Fruits of your choice (banana, blueberries, melon, kiwi, grapes, pear), chopped

INSTRUCTIONS:

1. You need popsicle molds/form. Place all fruits into the molds, leaving room for the sticks of a popsicle.

2. Pour in coconut water, but do not fill to top since the liquid will expand during the freezing.

3. Put them into the freezer until set.

NUTRITION:

calories 90fat 0g fiber 1g carbs 23gprotein 0

Pumpkin Walnut Custard

Prep. time: 5 min. Cooking time: 50 min. Servings: 4

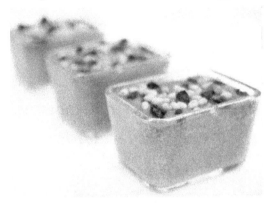

INGREDIENTS:

2 lb. 5 oz. pumpkin, baked and pureed

4 eggs

1 teaspoon cinnamon

1 teaspoon ginger

1/2 teaspoon nutmeg

1 can coconut milk

2 teaspoon vanilla bean powder

1 teaspoon pumpkin spice

¼ cup walnuts, chopped

Coconut oil

1 tablespoon ghee butter

Salt

INSTRUCTIONS:

1. Preheat oven to 350°F.Combine pumpkin, coconut milk, eggs, cinnamon, ginger, pumpkin spice, and nutmeg in a bowl. Add a pinch of salt.

2. Beat on high until all ingredients are well combined.

3. Grease 4 custard dishes with coconut oil. Pour in pumpkin mixture and bake in the oven for 30 minutes.

4. In a small bowl, combine walnuts, ghee butter, and vanilla bean powder. Microwave until melted and stir to combine.

5. Add topping to the center of custard and bake for another 20 minutes. Leave the custard to rest in the oven for a little bit to prevent it from cooling too quickly.

6. Put in the fridge for 4-5 hours to cool before serving. Top with walnuts.

NUTRITION:

calories 108 fat 7g fiber 3.3gcarbs 6.3g protein 5.9g

Sautéed Apples with Coconut Butter

Prep. time: 2 min. Cooking time: 10 min. Servings: 2-3

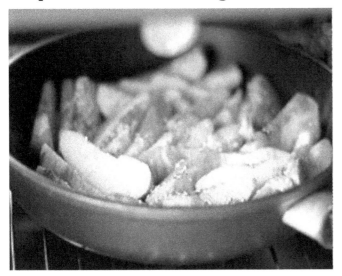

INGREDIENTS:

1 large apple, peeled and sliced

1 large pear, peeled and sliced

1-2 tablespoon coconut oil

2 teaspoon ground cinnamon

¼ teaspoon sea salt

3 tablespoon coconut butter, melted

INSTRUCTIONS:

1. Heat a medium nonstick skillet and add one tablespoon of the coconut oil

2. Once heated, add the apples and cook/stir one minute, then add the pears and combine.

3. Sprinkle the salt over the top and stir, continue to cook until softened, about 3 minutes, adding any extra coconut oil, and making heat lower if you need to.

4. Lower the heat and add the cinnamon over the fruits. Once the mixture is lightly browned, remove from the heat.

5. Microwave coconut butter in a glass for 5 sec until drippy but not too hot. Drizzle over apples and pears to serve. Enjoy!

NUTRITION:

calories 105fat 5g fiber 2.5g carbs 8g protein 2g

APPENDIX : RECIPES INDEX

CPSIA information can be obtained
at www.ICGtesting.com
Printed in the USA
BVHW051721280821
615417BV00004B/329